AF408218

Table of Contents

Introduction

A bland diet is a regimented diet option that a physician can use to help optimize his or her patient's overall health condition. The bland diet is a useful modality to employ when managing a patient with persistent gastrointestinal complaints, acid-peptic disease, excess gas formation or in certain postsurgical patients. The bland diet is sometimes referred to as a "low residue diet" or "soft diet." A bland diet is easier to break down and digest, therefore it gives rest to the gastrointestinal tract. It is also less acidic and causes fewer bowel movements.

The bland diet comprises of easily digestible foods that are soft-consistency, low-fiber, cooked, gentle to the gastrointestinal tract and usually non-spicy. A typical such diet includes, but is not limited to, low-fat dairy products, eggs, broth, pudding, fruit juices, cream of wheat, tofu, lean meat (skinless chicken, fish,...), bland vegetables (beet, bean, spinach, carrot,...), eggs, and tea. The diet also eliminates raw or uncooked foods.

What is avoided in this diet is typically anything "non-bland." This might include fried food, spices, seeds and nuts, acidic fruits (berries, grapes, oranges, lemons, limes,...), whole-grain bread (wheat, whole wheat pasta, cereal,...), fatty dairy food (whole milk, whipped cream, ice-cream,...), non-lean meat (beef, fried fish, chicken with attached skin), dressings and sauces, pickles, alcoholic beverages, strong cheeses, and vegetables that cause excesses flatulence (cabbage, cauliflower, onion, pepper...).

Avoiding some of these elements will change the taste of the foods and affect our pattern of eating. There is no easy answer or solution for this, but some changes and substitution might ease the difficulties. Some raw fruits can be substituted with pureed fruits and compotes; nuts can be replaced with nut butter, nutmeg with cinnamon,...; Broiling or mashing some foods, rather than frying them, might be quite helpful. Beverages are habitual and can easily be substituted. Fruit water or tea can replace soda, coffee, and energy drinks.

The bland diet is most useful in adjunct to lifestyle modifications for a patient that struggles with gastric or duodenal ulcers, gastroesophageal reflux disease (GERD), excess flatulence, food poisoning, gastroenteritis, traveler's diarrhea, inflammatory bowel disease, diverticulosis or heartburn. It may be utilized in a patient before colonic procedures like colonoscopy. [2] Also, the bland diet is a viable option after stomach and intestinal surgeries when the patient is being transitioned back to a regular diet.[3] The bland diet is mostly a temporary measure and not a permanent one.

Why eat a bland diet?

If you're dealing with gastrointestinal distress, eating a bland diet may help relieve heartburn, vomiting, diarrhea, and nausea. A bland diet can also be an effective way to treat peptic ulcers, especially when coupled with certain lifestyle changes, such as lessening stress.

To fit the bill, bland foods are typically soft in texture, lower in fiber, higher in pH, and mildly seasoned. These factors help prevent an increase in acid production, reflux, or other irritation to your digestive tract.

Despite its name, eating a bland diet can be as tasty as it is comforting to the gut. The best dietary approach for digestive symptoms is one that targets the root cause of your symptoms, so recommendations may vary from person to person. But generally, here's what you should eat, and what you should avoid.

What can I eat?

Everyone's needs are different, so you may want to discuss your dietary choices with your doctor or a dietitian. They can provide additional input based on your specific diagnosis and lifestyle.

Unless you have a preexisting food allergy or intolerance, commonly recommended foods on the bland diet include:

Low-fat dairy

Low-fat or fat-free milk, yogurt, and mildly flavored cheeses, such as cottage cheese, are all good options. Be careful, though. Lactose intolerance and milk protein intolerance are common reasons for GI discomfort in some people. And many experts recommend eliminating dairy to help treat peptic ulcers.

Certain vegetables

Vegetables you should eat include:

beets

carrots

green beans

peas

white or sweet potatoes

spinach

pumpkin

These vegetables can be purchased frozen, fresh, or canned. However, don't eat them raw. It's best to serve them steamed or boiled, with little to no butter or other type of fat.

Some people can tolerate lettuce and other salad greens in moderation. It's best to exclude vegetables that cause gas, such as those from the cruciferous family. These include broccoli, kale and Brussels sprouts, among others.

Low-fiber fruits

Cooked or canned fruits that aren't fibrous or seeded are generally approved for a bland diet. These include bananas and melon. Avocados may also be tolerated well, even though they're higher in fiber.

Processed grains

White bread products, seedless rye, and refined wheat products may be good choices. However, some people have worsened digestive symptoms when they eat gluten-containing grains.

If you do not have an intolerance to gluten, then you can also enjoy:

plain soda crackers

soft white pasta

cooked cereals, such as cream of wheat, processed oatmeal (not steel-cut or high-fiber), and farina

cold cereals that are low in sugar

Poultry, eggs, and fish

Lean protein sources are safe to eat as long as they're prepared with mild seasonings and little to no fat. These include:

skinless chicken

fish, such as salmon and trout

shellfish, such as shrimp, lobster, and crab

eggs

silken tofu

Other food items

Cream-based soups or clear broths are excellent choices, provided their ingredients are on the list of foods you can eat.

Chamomile tea, with or without honey, can be a soothing drink choice.

Dessert foods, such as vanilla pudding, marshmallows, and plain cookies should only be eaten sparingly because added sugar can worsen symptoms.

Creamy peanut butter, jelly, and jam without seeds are all good options for spreading on bread.

Many seasonings may be irritating to the stomach, but you can experiment with basil, parsley, salt, and other mild flavorings to determine which ones you can tolerate.

What should I avoid?

Foods affect everyone differently. Some people get heartburn and other gastric symptoms from tomato-based products, garlic, and caffeinated tea. Others can tolerate highly spiced foods, but have trouble digesting anything high in fat.

Your individual needs may vary, but in general, these foods should be avoided if you're following a bland diet:

High-fat dairy

High-fat dairy foods and strongly-flavored cheeses should be avoided. These include:

whole milk

whipped cream

ice cream

Monterey Jack cheese

bleu cheese

Roquefort cheese

Also, dairy triggers symptoms in some people, so avoid dairy altogether if this is you.

Certain vegetables

Some vegetables are notorious for producing gas. These include:

cruciferous types, such as Brussels sprouts, broccoli, and cauliflower

onion

garlic

peppers

cabbage

Tomatoes and tomato products are highly acidic and should be avoided.

Seeded and acidic fruit

In general, if fruit has skin or tiny seeds, it has too much fiber for a bland diet. Also, the acidity of some of the fruits may trigger heartburn in some people.

Fruits to avoid include:

all berries

grapes

prunes

oranges

lemons

limes

grapefruits

Most dried fruits and fruit juices should be eliminated, as well.

Whole grains

High-fiber, whole grain foods should be avoided if you are following a low-fiber or low-residue diet, which is sometimes recommended as part of a bland diet. Also, gluten may be a trigger for some people, so avoiding all forms of wheat, rye, and barley may be beneficial.

Avoid these:

sprouted wheat bread

grain breads

whole wheat pasta

any product with added fiber, such as cereal

Fatty meats, poultry, beans, and fish

Lentils and dried or canned beans of all types can generate gas. Beef, chicken with the skin on, and fried fish may also irritate your gut.

Avoid eating fatty, greasy, or fried protein sources of any kind, as well as processed deli meats. You should also avoid prepared foods, such as beef or chicken tacos, chili, or meat sauce.

Other food items

All types of alcoholic drinks can be irritating to the stomach. So can caffeinated beverages, such as coffee, tea, and soda.

Many dressings and sauces, such as mustard, ketchup, salad dressing, and horseradish, are best left on the shelf.

The following may also make your symptoms worse:

fatty desserts, such as cheesecake and dark chocolate

olives

popcorn

granola

nuts

BLAND DIET RECIPES

Juicy Roasted Chicken

Ingredient Checklist

1 (3 pound) whole chicken, giblets removed

1 teaspoon salt and black pepper to taste

1 tablespoon onion powder, or to taste

½ cup margarine, divided

1 stalk celery, leaves removed

Step 1

Preheat oven to 350 degrees F (175 degrees C).

Step 2

Place chicken in a roasting pan, and season generously inside and out with salt and pepper. Sprinkle inside and out with onion powder. Place 3 tablespoons margarine in the chicken cavity. Arrange dollops of the remaining margarine around the chicken's exterior. Cut the celery into 3 or 4 pieces, and place in the chicken cavity.

Step 3

Bake uncovered 1 hour and 15 minutes in the preheated oven, to a minimum internal temperature of 180 degrees F (82 degrees C). Remove from heat, and baste with melted margarine and drippings. Cover with aluminum foil, and allow to rest about 30 minutes before serving.

Spinach and Feta Pita Bake

Ingredient Checklist

1 (6 ounce) tub sun-dried tomato pesto

6 (6 inch) whole wheat pita breads

2 plum tomato (blank)s roma (plum) tomatoes, chopped

1 bunch spinach, rinsed and chopped

4 medium (blank)s fresh mushrooms, sliced

½ cup crumbled feta cheese

2 tablespoons grated Parmesan cheese

3 tablespoons olive oil

1 pinch ground black pepper to taste

Step 1

Preheat the oven to 350 degrees F (175 degrees C).

Step 2

Spread tomato pesto onto one side of each pita bread and place them pesto-side up on a baking sheet. Top pitas with tomatoes, spinach, mushrooms, feta cheese, and Parmesan cheese; drizzle with olive oil and season with pepper.

Step 3

Bake in the preheated oven until pita breads are crisp, about 12 minutes. Cut pitas into quarters.

Insalata Caprese II

Ingredient Checklist

4 large ripe tomatoes, sliced 1/4 inch thick

1 pound fresh mozzarella cheese, sliced 1/4 inch thick

⅓ cup fresh basil leaves

3 tablespoons extra virgin olive oil

½ teaspoon fine sea salt to taste

1 pinch freshly ground black pepper to taste

DirectionsInstructions Checklist

Step 1

On a large platter, alternate and overlap the tomato slices, mozzarella cheese slices, and basil leaves. Drizzle with olive oil. Season with sea salt and pepper.

Guacamole

Ingredient Checklist

3 avocado, NS as to Florida or Californias avocados - peeled, pitted, and mashed

1 lime, juiced

1 teaspoon salt

½ cup diced onion

3 tablespoons chopped fresh cilantro

2 plum tomato (blank)s roma (plum) tomatoes, diced

1 teaspoon minced garlic

1 pinch ground cayenne pepper

Step 1

In a medium bowl, mash together the avocados, lime juice, and salt. Mix in onion, cilantro, tomatoes, and garlic. Stir in cayenne pepper. Refrigerate 1 hour for best flavor, or serve immediately.

Taco Seasoning I

1 tablespoon chili powder

¼ teaspoon garlic powder

¼ teaspoon onion powder

¼ teaspoon crushed red pepper flakes

¼ teaspoon dried oregano

½ teaspoon paprika

1 ½ teaspoons ground cumin

1 teaspoon sea salt

1 teaspoon black pepper

Step 1

In a small bowl, mix together chili powder, garlic powder, onion powder, red pepper flakes, oregano, paprika, cumin, salt and pepper. Store in an airtight container.

Foolproof Rib Roast

Ingredient Checklist

1 (5 pound) standing beef rib roast

2 teaspoons salt

1 teaspoon ground black pepper

1 teaspoon garlic powder

Add All Ingredients To Shopping List

Step 1

Allow roast to stand at room temperature for at least 1 hour.

Step 2

Preheat the oven to 375 degrees F (190 degrees C). Combine the salt, pepper and garlic powder in a small cup. Place the roast on a rack in a roasting pan so that the fatty side is up and the rib side is on the bottom. Rub the seasoning onto the roast.

Step 3

Roast for 1 hour in the preheated oven. Turn the oven off and leave the roast inside. Do not open the door. Leave it in there for 3 hours. 30 to 40 minutes before serving, turn the oven back on at 375 degrees F (190 degrees C) to reheat the roast. The internal temperature should be at least 145 degrees F (62 degrees C). Remove from the oven and let rest for 10 minutes before carving into servings.

Marinated Grilled Shrimp

Ingredient Checklist

3 cloves garlic, minced

⅓ cup olive oil

¼ cup tomato sauce

2 tablespoons red wine vinegar

2 tablespoons chopped fresh basil

½ teaspoon salt

¼ teaspoon cayenne pepper

2 pounds fresh shrimp, peeled and deveined

6 eaches skewers

Step 1

In a large bowl, stir together the garlic, olive oil, tomato sauce, and red wine vinegar. Season with basil, salt, and cayenne pepper. Add shrimp to the bowl, and stir until evenly coated. Cover, and refrigerate for 30 minutes to 1 hour, stirring once or twice.

Step 2

Preheat grill for medium heat. Thread shrimp onto skewers, piercing once near the tail and once near the head. Discard marinade.

Step 3

Lightly oil grill grate. Cook shrimp on preheated grill for 2 to 3 minutes per side, or until opaque.

Rosemary Roasted Turkey

Ingredient Checklist

¾ cup olive oil

3 tablespoons minced garlic

2 tablespoons chopped fresh rosemary

1 tablespoon chopped fresh basil

1 tablespoon Italian seasoning

1 teaspoon ground black pepper

salt to taste

1 (12 pound) whole turkey

Step 1

Preheat oven to 325 degrees F (165 degrees C).

Step 2

In a small bowl, mix the olive oil, garlic, rosemary, basil, Italian seasoning, black pepper and salt. Set aside.

Step 3

Wash the turkey inside and out; pat dry. Remove any large fat deposits. Loosen the skin from the breast. This is done by slowly working your fingers between the breast and the skin. Work it loose to the end of the drumstick, being careful not to tear the skin.

Step 4

Using your hand, spread a generous amount of the rosemary mixture under the breast skin and down the thigh and leg. Rub the remainder of the rosemary mixture over the outside of the breast. Use toothpicks to seal skin over any exposed breast meat.

Step 5

Place the turkey on a rack in a roasting pan. Add about 1/4 inch of water to the bottom of the pan. Roast in the preheated oven 3 to 4 hours, or until the internal temperature of the bird reaches 180 degrees F (80 degrees C).

Simple Roasted Butternut Squash

Ingredient Checklist

1 butternut squash - peeled, seeded, and cut into 1-inch cubes

2 tablespoons olive oil

2 cloves garlic, minced

1 pinch salt and ground black pepper to taste

Step 1

Preheat oven to 400 degrees F (200 degrees C).

Step 2

Toss butternut s□uash with olive oil and garlic in a large bowl. Season with salt and black pepper. Arrange coated s□uash on a baking sheet.

Step 3

Roast in the preheated oven until s□uash is tender and lightly browned, 25 to 30 minutes.

Cajun Spice Mix

Ingredient Checklist

2 teaspoons salt

2 teaspoons garlic powder

2 ½ teaspoons paprika

1 teaspoon ground black pepper

1 teaspoon onion powder

1 teaspoon cayenne pepper

1 ¼ teaspoons dried oregano

1 ¼ teaspoons dried thyme

½ teaspoon red pepper flakes

 Step 1

Stir together salt, garlic powder, paprika, black pepper, onion powder, cayenne pepper, oregano, thyme, and red pepper flakes until evenly blended. Store in an airtight container.

Whole Chicken Slow Cooker Recipe

Ingredient Checklist

4 teaspoons salt, or to taste

2 teaspoons paprika

1 teaspoon cayenne pepper

1 teaspoon onion powder

1 teaspoon ground thyme

1 teaspoon ground white pepper

½ teaspoon garlic powder

½ teaspoon ground black pepper

1 whole whole chicken

Step 1

Mix salt, paprika, cayenne pepper, onion powder, thyme, white pepper, garlic powder, and black pepper together in a small bowl.

Step 2

Rub seasoning mixture over the entire chicken to evenly season. Put rubbed chicken into a large resealable plastic bag; refrigerate 8 hours to overnight.

Step 3

Remove chicken from bag and cook in slow cooker on Low until no longer pink at the bone and the juices run clear, 4 to 8 hours. An instant-read thermometer inserted into the thickest part of the thigh, near the bone should read 165 degrees F (74 degrees C).

Garlic Prime Rib

Ingredient Checklist

1 (10 pound) prime rib roast

10 cloves garlic, minced

2 tablespoons olive oil

2 teaspoons salt

2 teaspoons ground black pepper

2 teaspoons dried thyme

Step 1

Place the roast in a roasting pan with the fatty side up. In a small bowl, mix together the garlic, olive oil, salt, pepper and thyme. Spread the mixture over the fatty layer of the roast, and let the roast sit out until it is at room temperature, no longer than 1 hour.

Step 2

Preheat the oven to 500 degrees F (260 degrees C).

Step 3

Bake the roast for 20 minutes in the preheated oven, then reduce the temperature to 325 degrees F (165 degrees C), and continue roasting for an additional 60 to 75 minutes. The internal temperature of the roast should be at 135 degrees F (57 degrees C) for medium rare.

Step 4

Allow the roast to rest for 10 or 15 minutes before carving so the meat can retain its juices.

Roast Sticky Chicken-Rotisserie Style

Ingredient Checklist

4 teaspoons salt

2 teaspoons paprika

1 teaspoon onion powder

1 teaspoon dried thyme

1 teaspoon white pepper

½ teaspoon cayenne pepper

½ teaspoon black pepper

½ teaspoon garlic powder

2 medium (2-1/2" dia)s onions, quartered

2 (4 pound) whole chickens

Step 1

In a small bowl, mix together salt, paprika, onion powder, thyme, white pepper, black pepper, cayenne pepper, and garlic powder. Remove and discard giblets from chicken. Rinse chicken cavity, and pat dry with paper towel. Rub each chicken inside and out with spice mixture. Place 1 onion into the cavity of each chicken. Place chickens in a resealable bag or double wrap with plastic wrap. Refrigerate overnight, or at least 4 to 6 hours.

Step 2

Preheat oven to 250 degrees F (120 degrees C).

Step 3

Place chickens in a roasting pan. Bake uncovered for 5 hours, to a minimum internal temperature of 180 degrees F (85 degrees C). Let the chickens stand for 10 minutes before carving.

Ken's Perfect Hard Boiled Egg (And I Mean Perfect)

Ingredient Checklist

1 tablespoon salt

¼ cup distilled white vinegar

6 cups water

8 large eggs eggs

Step 1

Combine the salt, vinegar, and water in a large pot, and bring to a boil over high heat. Add the eggs one at a time, being careful not to crack them. Reduce the heat to a gentle boil, and cook for 14 minutes.

Step 2

Once the eggs have cooked, remove them from the hot water, and place into a container of ice water or cold, running water. Cool completely, about 15 minutes. Store in the refrigerator up to 1 week.

Roasted Asparagus Prosciutto and Egg

Ingredient Checklist

1 bunch fresh asparagus, trimmed

1 tablespoon extra-virgin olive oil

1 tablespoon olive oil

2 ounces minced prosciutto

1 pinch ground black pepper

1 teaspoon distilled white vinegar

1 pinch salt

4 medium (blank)s eggs

½ lemon, zested and juiced

1 pinch ground black pepper

Step 1

Preheat oven to 425 degrees F (220 degrees C). Place asparagus in a baking dish and drizzle with 1 tablespoon extra-virgin olive oil.

Step 2

Heat 1 tablespoon olive oil in a skillet over medium-low heat. Add prosciutto; cook, stirring, until golden and rendered, 3 to 4 minutes. Sprinkle prosciutto and oil over asparagus. Season with black pepper and toss to coat. Roast in the preheated oven for 10 minutes. Toss and return to oven until firm yet tender to the bite, 5 minutes.

Step 3

Fill a large saucepan with 2 to 3 inches of water and bring to a boil over high heat. Reduce heat to medium-low, pour in vinegar and pinch of salt. Crack an egg into a bowl then gently slip the egg into the water. Repeat with remaining eggs. Poach eggs until whites are firm and yolks have thickened but are not hard, 4 to 6 minutes. Remove eggs from water with a slotted spoon, dab on a kitchen towel to remove excess water, then transfer to a warm plate.

Step 4

Drizzle asparagus with lemon juice. Transfer asparagus to plates, top with poached egg and pinch of lemon zest. Season with black pepper and serve.

Best Marinara Sauce Yet

Ingredient Checklist

2 (14.5 ounce) cans stewed tomatoes

1 (6 ounce) can tomato paste

4 tablespoons chopped fresh parsley

1 clove garlic, minced

1 teaspoon dried oregano

1 teaspoon salt

¼ teaspoon ground black pepper

6 tablespoons olive oil

⅓ cup finely diced onion

½ cup white wine

DirectionsInstructions Checklist

Step 1

In a food processor place Italian tomatoes, tomato paste, chopped parsley, minced garlic, oregano, salt, and pepper. Blend until smooth.

Step 2

In a large skillet over medium heat saute the finely chopped onion in olive oil for 2 minutes. Add the blended tomato sauce and white wine.

Step 3

Simmer for 30 minutes, stirring occasionally.

Pico de Gallo

Ingredient Checklist

6 plum tomato (blank)s roma (plum) tomatoes, diced

½ red onion, minced

3 tablespoons chopped fresh cilantro

½ jalapeno pepper, seeded and minced

½ lime, juiced

1 clove garlic, minced

1 pinch garlic powder

1 pinch ground cumin, or to taste

1 pinch salt and ground black pepper to taste

Add All Ingredients To Shopping List

Step 1

Stir the tomatoes, onion, cilantro, jalapeno pepper, lime juice, garlic, garlic powder, cumin, salt, and pepper together in a bowl. Refrigerate at least 3 hours before serving.

Grilled Asparagus

Ingredient Checklist

1 pound fresh asparagus spears, trimmed

1 tablespoon olive oil

1 pinch salt and pepper to taste

Step 1

Preheat grill for high heat.

Step 2

Lightly coat the asparagus spears with olive oil. Season with salt and pepper to taste.

Step 3

Grill over high heat for 2 to 3 minutes, or to desired tenderness.

Roasted Okra

Ingredient Checklist

18 eaches fresh okra pods, sliced 1/3 inch thick

1 tablespoon olive oil

2 teaspoons kosher salt, or to taste

2 teaspoons black pepper, or to taste

Add All Ingredients To Shopping List

Step 1

Preheat an oven to 425 degrees F (220 degrees C).

Step 2

Arrange the okra slices in one layer on a foil lined cookie sheet. Drizzle with olive oil and sprinkle with salt and pepper. Bake in the preheated oven for 10 to 15 minutes.

WEIGHT LOSS AND MANGING DIABETS RECIPES

Slow Cooker Seafood Ramen

Ingredients:

64 oz broth (seafood, vegetable, or chicken

4–6 oz ramen

1 lb seafood

2 green onions, sliced

2 tbsp low-sodium soy sauce

2 tbsp rice vinegar

2 garlic cloves, minced

1/4 cup kale, chopped

1/2 lb tomatoes, sliced

1/4 tsp sesame oil

1 tsp salt

1/4 tsp pepper

1/8 tsp red pepper flakes

Directions:

Add all ingredients except the seafood, kale and ramen to the slow cooker. Stir to mix well.

Cook on high for 2-3 hours, or low for 4-6 hours.

Add seafood, kale & ramen and cook for an additional 15-30 minutes.

Per Serving: 250 calories, 2.7 g fat (0.3 g sat), 29.5 g protein, 27 g carb, 2588.3 mg sodium, 3.9 g sugars, 1.7 g fiber

Turkey Carrot Mushroom Dumplings

Ingredients:

3/4 c. carrots finely julienned

1 lb ground turkey

1/2 c. mushrooms finely chopped

2 tsp soy sauce

1 tsp rice wine

1 tsp sesame oil

1/2 tsp onion powder

1/8 tsp salt

2 tsp cornstarch

30 dumpling wrappers

Directions:

Put carrots in a microwavable bowl and cover with water. Cook until tender, about 3 minutes depending on how finely shredded the carrots are. Drain and let cool.

In a large bowl, mix together cooked carrots, turkey, mushrooms, soy sauce, rice wine, sesame oil, onion powder, salt and cornstarch. Stir together until well combined.

Spoon a well rounded teaspoon of filling onto a dumpling wrapper. Seal filling with wrapper. Wrap remaining dumplings.

Bring water to boil in the bottom of the steamer pot. Place dumplings in a parchment paper lined steamer. Steam 15 minutes until cooked through.

Per serving: 48 calories, 1 g fat (0 g sat), 3 g protein, 4 g carb, 87 mg sodium

Slow Grilled Chinese Char Siu Chicken

Ingredients:

1/4 c. organic brown sugar

1/4 c. raw honey

1/4 c. organic ketchup

1/4 c. gluten-free soy sauce

3 Tbsp beet powder

2 Tbsp rice vinegar

1 Tbsp gluten-free hoisin sauce

1/2 tsp Chinese five-spice powder

Sea salt and freshly ground black pepper to taste

2 1/2 lbs boneless skinless chicken thighs

Cooking oil spray

Directions:

In a large bowl, mix together brown sugar, honey, ketchup, soy sauce, beet powder, vinegar, hoisin sauce, five-spice powder, salt and pepper.

Add chicken and toss well, coating all the pieces well; cover and refrigerate for two days to marinate.

Heat grill; spray cooking oil on grates; grill chicken until cooked through, about 10 minutes per side.

Per serving: 328 calories, 8 g fat (2 g sat), 38 g protein, 25 g carb, 845 mg sodium, 24 g sugars, 1 g fiber

Creamy Kabocha Squash and Roasted Red Pepper Pasta

Ingredients:

1/2 c. raw cashews

1 small kabocha squash

1 head of garlic

1/3 cauliflower, cut into large florets

1/2 medium onion (roughly chopped)

1 stalk celery, roughly chopped

1 medium carrot, roughly chopped

1/4 c. roasted red peppers, drained

2 Tbsp nutritional yeast

Optional: A pinch red pepper flakes

2 to 3 c. vegetable broth (or as needed)

Salt and black pepper, to taste

1/2 to 3/4 c. fresh basil (unpacked), sliced

2 lb gluten-free spaghetti noodles (or pasta of your choice)

Serve with:

Vegan parmesan cheese (optional)

Fresh basil, sliced

Black pepper

Directions:

Soak the cashews in water overnight. If you do not have time to, you can also bring a small pot of water to a boil, remove it from heat and add in the cashews. Allow them to soak until you blend the sauce together (which will be about 1 hour).

Preheat the oven to 400°F and position the rack to the middle of the oven. Line a baking sheet with parchment paper or a silicone mat. Wash and dry the kabocha squash, place it (whole) on the baking sheet and into the oven for 18-20 minutes. Remove the pan from the oven and cool until the squash is easy to handle. If the stem of it is protruding, use a knife to carefully remove it. Slice the squash in half vertically, then scoop out the seeds and fiber using a spoon. Slice the squash into 1-inch wedges, trying to keep the slices uniform for even cooking. Place 6 or 7 the slices of the cooked squash (roughly 1 1/2 cups) onto your lined baking sheet. The remaining kabocha squash can be cooked on an additional baking sheet with the same baking time and directions below. It can be stored in the fridge in an airtight container for up to a week.

Using your hands, remove loose skin from the outside of the head of garlic. With a sharp knife, cut 1/4"-inch off the top of the garlic, or enough to expose the tops of the cloves. Place the garlic head (cut side down) onto the baking sheet along with the cauliflower florets, onions, celery, and carrots. Sprinkle with salt and pepper and place back into the oven for 40 minutes, flipping/mixing halfway through.

10 minutes before the vegetables are done, prepare the pasta.

Once you have removed the baking sheet from the oven, allow the veggies to cool until easily handled and then use a knife to carefully remove the skin from the kabocha and add it into a high speed blender. You can discard this or snack on it as you continue cooking. Using you hands, squeeze the soften garlic cloves out of the head and into the blender, along with the soaked cashews (drained), the remaining vegetables on the baking sheet, the roasted red peppers, nutritional yeast, red pepper flakes, 2 cups of vegetable broth plus salt and pepper as desired. Blend until smooth, adding as much of the additional 1 cup of vegetable broth as needed to thin out the sauce. Adjust seasonings to taste and then add in the sliced basil. Pulse the basil in until well combined (do not blend it as it will turn the sauce a weird color).

Drain the pasta, add it back into the pot and pour over the sauce. Mix until well combined.

Serve with a sprinkle of fresh parmesan, basil and black pepper. Enjoy!

Per serving: 501 calories, 5.9 g fat (0 g sat), 17.8 g protein, 93.4 g carb, 56.3 mg sodium, 5.8 g sugars

Loaded Cauliflower

Ingredients:

1.25 lb cauliflower head, cut into florets

6 green onion, chopped into the green and white parts

2 tbsp butter

3 garlic cloves, minced

2 oz cream cheese

1/2 tsp sea salt

1/4 tsp black pepper

1.5 tsp ranch seasoning Mix, optional

3/4 c. organic heavy whipping cream

2 c. cheddar cheese, grated

4 slices sugar-free bacon, crumbled

Olive oil for roasting the cauliflower

Dollops of sour cream, optional

Directions:

Preheat the oven to 425 degrees.

Toss the cauliflower with ~2 Tbsp of olive oil then add it to a baking sheet. Roast the cauliflower on a baking sheet for 25 minutes. The cauliflower will get tender and some parts will brown up.

While the cauliflower is roasting, make the cheese sauce: Add butter, the white parts of the green onions, and the garlic cloves to a skillet on medium heat. Sauté until the onions are translucent (~3 minutes).

Add heavy cream, cream cheese, salt, ranch seasoning (if you're using it), and pepper to the skillet with the onions, garlic and butter. Turn the heat to medium low and continue to cook until the cream cheese is melted. Stir in 1.5 cups of the cheddar cheese to finish the cheese sauce.

Mix the cheese sauce and the roasted cauliflower, then add it to a baking dish. Top it with the remaining cheddar cheese and roast for an additional 20 minutes, or until the cauliflower is tender.

Top the baked cauliflower, with some dollops of sour cream, the green parts of the green onions, and the crumbled bacon.

Per serving: 315 calories, 28 g fat (17 g sat), 11 g protein, 5 g carb, 587 mg sodium, 2 g sugars, 1 g fiber

Easy Creamy Cajun Shrimp Pasta

Ingredients:

8 oz linguine pasta

2 tsp olive oil Divided into 1 teaspoon servings.

1 lb raw shrimp, deveined and shells removed.

1 Tbsp cajun seasoning divided into 1/2 Tbsp servings. You can also use creole seasoning.

4 oz andouille sausage Sliced into 1 inch pieces. You can use more if you like.

1/2 c. chopped red peppers

1/2 c. chopped green peppers

1/2 c. chopped yellow or white onions

1 c. fire roasted diced tomatoes Drained from a can.

1 Tbsp butter

1/2 c. heavy whipping cream

1/2 c. unsweetened almond milk

4 oz cream cheese Cut into chunks.

1/2 c. shredded Parmesan Reggiano Cheese

Directions

Cook the pasta as per package instructions.

Place the shrimp in a bowl along with 1/2 Tbsp of cajun or creole seasoning. Mix to ensure the shrimp is fully coated.

Heat a skillet or pan on medium high heat. I use a cast iron skillet. Add 1 teaspoon of olive oil to the pan.

When hot, add the shrimp to the pan. Cook for 2-3 minutes on each side until it turns bright pink. Remove the shrimp and set aside.

Add an additional teaspoon of olive oil to the pan along with the chopped sausage, onions, green peppers, and red peppers.

Saute for 3-4 minutes until the vegetables are soft and the onions are translucent and fragrant. Remove the vegetables from the pan and set aside.

Reduce the heat on the pan to medium. Add the butter to the pan and allow it to melt.

Add in the heavy cream, almond milk, cream cheese, the remaining 1/2 tablespoon of cajun or creole seasoning, and parmesan reggiano cheese.

Continue to stir the sauce until all of the cheese has fully melted. The cream cheese may take some time to melt. Add in the fire roasted tomatoes and stir. Allow the mixture to cook for 2 minutes.

Add the shrimp, sausage, vegetables, and pasta to the pan and stir. Allow the pasta to cook for 4-5 minutes until combined. Serve.

Per serving: 384 calories, 28 g fat, 7 g protein, 22 g carb

Healthy Chicken Taco Soup

Ingredients:

½ Tbsp avocado or coconut oil

1 small yellow onion, diced

1 small red bell pepper, diced

1 small green bell pepper, diced

5 cloves garlic, minced

1 lb boneless, skinless chicken breast

1 1/2 tsp salt (plus more to taste)

1 tsp dried oregano

1 tsp chipotle powder

1 tsp paprika

2 tsp cumin

¼ tsp black pepper

1 – 15 oz can fire roasted diced tomatoes

2 – 4.5 oz cans green chilies

¼ c. fresh lime juice

32 oz chicken broth

Cilantro, for serving

Diced red onion, for serving

Lime wedges, for serving

Directions:

Heat a large pot over medium-high heat. Once hot, add in the avocado or coconut oil. Next, add the peppers, onion, and garlic to the pot. Saute for 3-4 minutes until the onions start to become translucent.

Add the chicken breast, canned tomatoes, canned green chilies, spices, lime juice, and chicken broth to the pot. Stir until well combined. Bring the soup to a rolling boil and then reduce the heat to a simmer. Allow the soup to simmer for 30 minutes or until the chicken is tender and easy to shred.

Transfer the chicken breast from the soup to a small bowl. Use two forks to shred the meat. Add the chicken back to the soup and stir until well combined. Serve the soup with fresh cilantro, diced red onion, and fresh lime wedges. Enjoy!

Per serving: 258 calories, 6.1 g fat (1 g sat), 30 g protein, 22.7 g carb, 1960.9 mg sodium, 10.1 g sugars, 5.1 g fiber

Quick and Easy Mongolian Beef

Ingredients:

1 lb flank steak thinly sliced against the grain

2 Tbsp cornstarch

2-4 Tbsp canola oil

1 yellow onion sliced

2 green onions chopped, green and white parts separated

4 garlic cloves chopped

1- inch ginger chopped

¼ c. low sodium soy sauce

¼ c. water

1 Tbsp hoisin sauce

3 Tbsp brown sugar

Salt to taste

Directions:

Cover the flank steak with cornstarch, making sure each piece is covered. Set aside.

Heat the canola oil in a large skillet over medium-high heat. Once the oil is hot, add the flank steak to the frying pan in a single layer, making sure that the pieces are not touching. Cook for 1-2 minutes per side until each side is browned. Cook in batches until all the flank steak is cooked. Set aside.

Add sliced yellow onion, whites of green onions, garlic, and ginger to the skillet and stir fry for about 3 minutes, until the onions are slightly softened but still have a little crunch. Add soy sauce, water, hoisin sauce, and brown sugar and stir. Add steak back to the pan along with the green parts of the onions. Remove from heat and serve.

Per serving: 303 calories, 13 g fat (3 g sat), 26 g protein, 20 g carb, 670 mg sodium, 11 g sugars, 1 g fiber

Caribbean Steamed Fish

Ingredients:

2 lbs fish (porgy or snapper), cleaned and scaled

Juice of 1 lime

½ tsp black pepper

1 tsp salt

3 cloves garlic – 2 sliced and 1 crushed

About 15 sprigs thyme

½ Tbsp butter

½ Tbsp oil

2 carrots, thinly sliced

1 red pepper, thinly sliced

1 green pepper, thinly sliced

1 onion, thinly sliced

12 okra, ends cut off

1 hot pepper (scotch bonnet, habanero or wiri wiri), seeds removed

1 ½ cup water

Directions:

Season the fish with lime juice, crushed garlic, black pepper, salt and half of the thyme and set aside.

In a large, wide heavy bottom pot over medium heat, add oil and butter. When butter has melted, sauté carrots, red and green pepper, and onion until it has softened, about 5 minutes.

Add garlic slices and pepper and cook for just a minute or two. Add water and bring to a boil. Add fish to the pot. Spoon some of the vegetables on top of the fish. Add okra and the rest of the thyme.

Cover the pot and lower the heat to simmer then cook for 15 minutes until the fish is done. Remove from heat and serve.

Per serving: 378 calories, 7.4 g fat (1.2 g sat), 60.5 g protein, 13.1 g carb, 794 mg sodium, 5.5 g sugars, 3.3 g fiber

Corn Chowder Con Chile Poblano

Ingredients:

2 Tbsp vegetable oil

1 poblano pepper without seeds and thinly sliced

1 medium onion sliced

2 cloves of garlic roughly chopped

5 corn husks

4 medium potatoes cubed

1 tsp of salt

To serve:

Corn kernels

Pumpkin seeds

Cilantro microgreens or chopped cilantro

Olive oil

Freshly ground pepper

Directions:

In a large pot add the oil and the sliced poblano chile. Leave it there until it begins to soften. Add the onion and garlic. Leave for five more minutes or until you see that the onion is translucent.

Add the corn kernels, potatoes, salt and cover with water, add the salt and cover. Leave for 10-15 minutes or until the vegetables are cooked.

With a ladle, add about one-third of the vegetables and liquid into the container of a blender. Blend until fully liquefied and well integrated. Return to the pot with the rest of the vegetables. If you need more liquid, add a little more water. Check for seasoning and adjust if necessary.

Serve with a drizzle of olive oil, pumpkin seeds, corn kernels, sprouts or chopped cilantro. Finish with sea salt and pepper.

Per serving: 135 calories, 4 g fat (3 g sat), 4 g protein, 20 g carb, 403 mg sodium, 1 g sugars, 4 g fiber

Crispy Potato Tacos

Ingredients:

12 corn tortillas

1 c. mashed potatoes

4 Tbsp of vegetable oil or avocado oil

4 long wooden skewers

To serve:

Thinly sliced romaine lettuce or green cabbage

Radishes thinly sliced

Cilantro

Guacamole

Salsa verde

Directions:

Heat tortillas on a skillet for 10-15 seconds to make them pliable.

Put a spoonful of mashed potatoes in the center of each tortilla and spread it along the tortilla. Roll the tortilla and put it on a long skewer. Repeat until you put three or four tacos on the skewer.

Repeat with all the tortillas.

In a frying pan over high heat put a tablespoon of oil and put three or four tacos, leave until golden brown, three to five minutes, turn and brown on the other side.

Take out the tacos and put in a dish with a paper towel to absorb the excess oil.

Repeat until all the tacos are done.

To serve, put the crispy potato tacos on a plate and finish with the toppings. Enjoy immediately.

Per serving: 347 calories, 16 g fat (2 g sat), 6 g protein, 47 g carb, 51 mg sodium, 1 g sugars, 6 g fiber

Black Garlic, Sesame and Shitake Cod

Ingredients:

2 Alaskan Cod filets, frozen

1 clove black garlic

2 Tbsp olive oil

1 tsp sesame seeds

1/2 c. dried shiitake, rehydrated

Directions:

Preheat your oven to 450F.

Rinse frozen fish, pat dry with a paper towel, and place on a non-stick pan.

In a small bowl, place black garlic and warm in the microwave for 10 seconds.

Mash the garlic clove and add olive oil and sesame seeds.

Brush this mixture on frozen filets and sprinkle the mushrooms around the fish.

Place in the oven for 12-15 minutes, depending on the thickness of the fish. If your filets are on the thick side, flip halfway through cooking.

Serve alongside rice, your favorite salad, or whole grain.

Per serving: 241 calories, 15.8 g fat (2.1 g sat), 20.9 g protein, 6.1 g carb, 72 mg sodium, 1.3 g sugars, 1 g fiber

Shrimp Lettuce Wraps

Ingredients:

1 head butter lettuce or romaine lettuce hearts

¼ c. low-sodium chicken broth

1 Tbsp hoisin sauce

½ Tbsp low-sodium soy sauce

1 tsp rice vinegar

¼ tsp Asian sesame oil

1 1/2 tsp chili garlic sauce

½ tsp cornstarch

1 Tbsp canola or avocado oil divided

30 grams cashews little less than ¼ cup, coarsely chopped

6 oz shrimp deveined & cut into small cubes

1 large garlic clove minced

1/2 large red bell pepper seeded and diced

3 green onions the white and green parts, sliced

⅛ c. chopped cilantro

1 carrot shredded or cut into thin strips

Directions:

Divide the lettuce into leaves and set aside.

In a small bowl, whisk together the chicken broth, hoisin sauce, soy sauce, rice vinegar, sesame oil, chili garlic sauce, and cornstarch. Set aside.

In a medium skillet, heat ½ Tbsp canola or avocado oil over medium-high heat until almost smoking.

Add the shrimp and stir-fry until browned. About 2 minutes. Transfer the shrimp to a plate and discard any juices from the pan.

In the same skillet, heat the other ½ tablespoon of oil over medium-high heat.

Add the garlic, bell pepper, green onions, and carrots.

Stir fry until tender-crisp, about 2 minutes.

Return the shrimp to the pan and add the cashews and cilantro. Add the soy-sauce mixture and stir-fry until the shrimp is thoroughly cooked. About 3 minutes.

Spoon the shrimp mixture evenly onto lettuce leaves.

Per serving: 269 calories, 14 g fat (2 g sat), 26 g protein, 17 g carb, 753 mg sodium, 7 g sugars, 3 g fiber

Baked Salmon Cake Balls With Rosemary Aioli

Ingredients:

2 lbs wild salmon fillets

1 tsp sea salt

1 tsp black pepper

1/2 medium purple onion, chopped

1/2 c. organic spinach, chopped

1/2 red bell pepper, diced

1/2 yellow red pepper, diced

1 small jalapeño, diced

2/3 c. breadcrumbs

1-2 Tbsps Old Bay seasoning

1/2 c. fresh parsley, chopped

1/3 c. vegan Mayo

1/2 c. dijon mustard

1 large organic egg, room temp.

4 Tbsps lemon juice

1-2 Tbsps sriracha sauce

1/2 c. vegan mayo

4 tsp lemon juice

2 garlic cloves, crushed + minced

1/4 tsp sea salt

2 sprigs fresh rosemary, chopped

Directions:

First, preheat the oven to 400 degrees Fahrenheit.

Season salmon with sea salt + black pepper and roast on a baking sheet (lined with parchment paper) for about 20 minutes, or until cooked through.

Once cooked, remove from the oven and set aside while it cools for 5 minutes before shredding or flaking into medium chunks.

Meanwhile, add onions, bell peppers, jalapeños, spinach, old bay seasoning, breadcrumbs, parsley, mayo, dijon mustard, egg, sriracha and lemon juice to a large bowl. Then add shredded salmon and mix all ingredients together, using your hands.

Scoop about 2 Tbsps of batter and form into a ball with your hands and line on a baking sheet (lined with parchment paper). Repeat until all batter is used.

Bake salmon balls for 15-20 minutes, or until slightly crisp and golden brown.

Combine vegan mayo, lemon juice, garlic cloves, sea salt, and rosemary in a medium bowl and whisk together thoroughly. Refrigerate for aioli until ready to use.

Per serving: 173 calories, 6.7 g fat (1.6 g sat), 20.5 g protein, 8.6 g carb, 6011 mg sodium, 3.3 g sugars, 1.2 g fiber

Crispy Baked Falafel

Ingredients:

1 c. dried chickpeas, soaked in water overnight

1/2 c. fresh parsley

1/2 medium onion chopped

3 garlic cloves chopped

1 tsp cumin

1 tsp coriander

1/4 tsp black pepper

1 tsp salt

1/4 c. vegetable oil

Directions:

Preheat the oven to 400F.

Once the chickpeas are done soaking, drain them and rinse with fresh water.

Add the soaked chickpeas, parsley, onion, garlic, spices, pepper and salt to a food processor. Pulse a few times, until you have a consistent, coarse texture.

Create 10-12 small falafel balls with your hands.

In a medium pan, heat the vegetable oil on the stovetop, and add the falafel balls. I recommend you do this in 2 batches.

Cook the falafel balls in the oil for 2 minutes on each side, using a spatula to carefully flip over. Once done, add them to a parchment paper-lined baking dish.

Once all the falafels are cooked on the pan and added to the baking dish, drizzle the remaining oil from the pan onto the falafels, and bake for 20 minutes or until browned and crisp. Flip halfway with a spatula.

Enjoy with pita, greens, rice, or your favorite pairings.

Per serving: 128 calories, 6.7 g fat (1.2 g sat), 4.1 g protein, 13 g carb, 261 mg sodium, 2.4 g sugars, 3.7 g fiber

Easy Vegetable Stirfry With Peanut Sauce

Ingredients:

Peanut Sauce:

1 Tbsp sesame oil

1/2 tsp ground ginger (1 tbsp fresh)

1/4 tsp garlic powder (2 cloves)

1/2 c. smooth unsweetened peanut butter

3 Tbsp low sodium soy sauce

2 Tbsp freshly squeezed lime juice

2 Tbsp maple syrup

2 Tbsp fresh lime juice

1 Tbsp rice vinegar

1/4 cc-1/3 cc water as needed

Optional: Sriracha, to taste

Stirfy:

6 oz dried noodles of choice (see notes)

1 Tbsp cooking oil of choice

3 cloves garlic, finely minced

2 Tbsp green onions sliced

1 Tbsp freshly grated ginger

1/3 c. shredded red cabbage

4 oz crimini mushrooms, sliced

1 medium carrot, thinly sliced

1 medium red bell pepper, thinly sliced

1 c. broccoli

2 large handfuls fresh baby spinach

Garnish:

Cilantro, finely chopped

Green onions, sliced

Toasted sesame seeds or crushed peanuts

1 large lime, sliced

Directions:

Prepare the peanut sauce: In a small pot over medium-low, add in the sesame oil, garlic and ginger. Cook until fragrant, about 2 minutes. Add in the remaining ingredients for the peanut sauce and whisk together until uniform. Allow the mixture to come to a low simmer and then remove from heat and set aside.

Prepare the noodles according to the package directions. Once the noodles are cooked, drain them, rinse under cold water, add them back into the cooking pot and toss them with about 1 teaspoon of sesame oil to prevent sticking.

In the meantime, set a large wok over medium heat. Add in the cooking oil along with the garlic, green onions and ginger. Sauté, stirring often, for 3 minutes or until fragrant.

Next add in the cabbage, mushrooms, carrots, bell pepper and broccoli. Cook for an additional 4 minutes.

Once the vegetables have cooked, add in the spinach, peanut sauce and cooked noodles. Mix until everything is well combined and cook for 1-2 minutes more, or until everything is warmed through.

Serve with a garnish of cilantro, green and toasted sesame seeds, plus an extra wedge of lime on the side. Enjoy!

Per serving: 388 calories, 19.7 g fat, 8.7 g protein, 47 g carb, 294.5 mg sodium, 11.6 g sugars

Conclusion

In essence, traditional foods are those whole and ancient foods that have been eaten for centuries and even millennium. They are the foods that your great-great-great-great-great grandmother and grandfather would have eaten. They are simple, naturally grown or raised, nutrient-dense, thoughtfully prepared. They are not fads (in fact, they tend to go in direct opposition to most conventional nutritional advice these days).

TRADITIONAL FOODS ARE :

Foods in their original form, as they were Created-not modernized, not processed, not packaged.

Foods that have a long history of supporting good health.

Foods that are whole and nutrient-dense.

Foods that are simple and basic: meat and poultry, eggs, whole grains, fish, beans and legumes, vegetables, fruit, nuts and seeds, dairy, fats.

TRADITIONAL FOODS AREN'T :

A one-size fits all diet (rather it has to do with a healthful variety of foods that are local to you, so if you live on the coast you may eat more fish, but if you live in a fertile valley you may eat plenty of raw dairy and vegetables).

The so-call"health foods" that you'll find with bold labels on the store shelves.

Low-fat, low-cholesterol, vegetarian or vegan.

Boring, bland, undesirable. (Quite the opposite- I think that once you get accustomed to them, you'll find that traditional foods taste incredible and are easy to love!)